7-DAYS BODY DETOX DIET

Revitalize your body: unlock vitality, shed toxins, heal and energy your life with proven strategies for optimal health and well-being

Odesa Mulan

Table of Contents

COPYRIGHT © 2023

CHAPTER ONE

Introduction to the 7-Day Body Detox Diet

In a world where wellness trends constantly evolve, the 7-Day Body Detox Diet has gained significant traction as a method for rebooting the body and achieving optimal health. This dietary approach is founded on the principle of eliminating toxins from the body, which proponents argue can lead to a wide range of health benefits, including increased energy levels, improved digestion, clearer skin, and weight loss. However, like any dietary regimen, it's essential to understand the science behind it, its potential benefits and risks, and how to approach it effectively.

Understanding the Concept of Detoxification

Detoxification, in the context of the body, refers to the process of eliminating or neutralizing toxins that accumulate within the body. These toxins can originate from various sources, including environmental pollutants, processed foods, alcohol, medications, and metabolic byproducts. The body has its natural detoxification mechanisms primarily carried out by the liver, kidneys, lungs, skin, and lymphatic system. However, proponents of detox diets argue that these mechanisms can become overwhelmed in our modern, toxin-laden environment, leading to the need for dietary interventions to support detoxification.

The Basis of the 7-Day Body Detox Diet

The 7-Day Body Detox Diet is designed to support the body's natural detoxification processes by providing it with nutrient-dense foods that promote liver function, enhance elimination pathways, and reduce exposure to toxins. Typically, this diet involves eliminating processed foods, refined sugars, caffeine, alcohol, and potentially allergenic foods for a period of seven days. Instead, the diet focuses on consuming whole foods such as fruits, vegetables, lean proteins, whole grains, nuts, seeds, and plenty of water.

Key Components of the 7-Day Body Detox Diet

1. **Hydration**: Adequate hydration is essential for supporting the body's detoxification processes. Water helps flush out toxins through urine and sweat and supports optimal liver and kidney function. In addition to water, herbal teas and fresh juices may also be included to provide hydration and additional nutrients.

2. **Whole Foods**: The foundation of the 7-Day Body Detox Diet is whole, minimally processed foods that are rich in vitamins, minerals, antioxidants, and fiber. These include fruits, vegetables, legumes, whole grains, nuts, and seeds. These foods provide essential nutrients that support detoxification pathways and overall health.

3. **Liver Support**: Certain foods and nutrients are believed to support liver function, which plays a central role in

detoxification. These include cruciferous vegetables (such as broccoli, cabbage, and kale), which contain compounds like glucosinolates and sulforaphane that support liver detoxification enzymes. Other liver-supportive foods include garlic, onions, turmeric, and green tea.

4. **Elimination of Processed Foods and Allergens**: Processed foods, refined sugars, artificial additives, and potential allergens are often eliminated during the detox period to reduce the body's exposure to toxins and potential allergens. This allows the digestive system to rest and repair while focusing on nutrient-dense whole foods.

5. **Mindful Eating**: The 7-Day Body Detox Diet emphasizes mindful eating practices, such as chewing food thoroughly, eating slowly, and paying attention to hunger and satiety cues. This approach promotes digestion, nutrient absorption, and overall awareness of food choices.

Potential Benefits of the 7-Day Body Detox Diet

Proponents of the 7-Day Body Detox Diet claim a variety of potential benefits, including:

1. **Increased Energy Levels**: By eliminating processed foods and focusing on nutrient-dense whole foods, proponents argue that individuals may experience increased energy levels and improved vitality.

2. **Improved Digestion**: The emphasis on whole foods and hydration may support digestive health, reduce bloating and discomfort, and promote regular bowel movements.

3. **Clearer Skin**: Some proponents suggest that removing potential skin irritants such as processed foods and allergens may lead to clearer, healthier skin.

4. **Weight Loss**: While not the primary focus, some individuals may experience weight loss during the detox period due to reduced calorie intake, increased consumption of whole foods, and potential elimination of water retention.

5. **Reduced Inflammation**: Whole foods and anti-inflammatory nutrients found in fruits, vegetables, and herbs may help reduce inflammation in the body, leading to improved overall health.

Criticism and Controversy

Despite its popularity, the 7-Day Body Detox Diet has faced criticism and controversy from some health experts and nutritionists.

1. **Lack of Scientific Evidence**: Critics argue that there is limited scientific evidence to support the efficacy of detox diets in eliminating toxins from the body or providing significant health benefits beyond what a balanced diet already offers.

2. **Potential Nutrient Deficiencies**: Depending on the specific guidelines of the detox diet, individuals may not consume an adequate amount of essential nutrients such as protein, fat, vitamins, and minerals, leading to potential nutrient deficiencies.

3. **Potential for Disordered Eating**: Detox diets with strict rules and limited food choices may promote unhealthy attitudes towards food, leading to disordered eating patterns or even the development of eating disorders in susceptible individuals.

4. **Short-Term Results**: While individuals may experience short-term benefits such as weight loss or increased energy levels during the detox period, these effects may not be sustainable in the long term without adopting permanent lifestyle changes.

Conclusion

The 7-Day Body Detox Diet is a popular dietary approach aimed at supporting the body's natural detoxification processes and promoting overall health and well-being. While proponents claim various benefits, including increased energy, improved digestion, and clearer skin, critics argue that the scientific evidence supporting these claims is limited. Furthermore, detox diets may pose risks such as potential nutrient deficiencies and the promotion of disordered eating patterns. As with any dietary regimen, it's essential to approach the 7-Day Body Detox Diet with caution, considering individual health needs and consulting with a healthcare professional before making significant changes to one's diet.

CHAPTER TWO

Understanding the Importance of Detoxification for Health

Detoxification, the process by which the body eliminates toxins, is essential for maintaining optimal health and well-being. In today's world, we are constantly exposed to environmental pollutants, chemicals in our food and water, and other toxins that can accumulate in the body over time. Understanding the importance of detoxification for health involves examining the body's natural detoxification mechanisms, the potential consequences of toxin accumulation, and how supporting detoxification can promote overall wellness.

The Body's Natural Detoxification Mechanisms

The human body has sophisticated mechanisms in place to neutralize and eliminate toxins. These mechanisms primarily involve the liver, kidneys, lungs, skin, and lymphatic system.

1. **Liver**: The liver is the body's primary detoxification organ. It processes toxins, breaking them down into less harmful substances that can be excreted from the body. The liver also produces enzymes that facilitate detoxification reactions.

2. **Kidneys**: The kidneys filter waste products and toxins from the blood, which are then excreted in urine. Proper

hydration is essential for supporting kidney function and promoting the elimination of toxins through urine.

3. **Lungs**: The lungs play a role in detoxification by eliminating volatile toxins through exhalation. Breathing clean air and avoiding exposure to pollutants can support lung health and detoxification.

4. **Skin**: The skin is the body's largest organ and plays a role in detoxification through sweating. Sweating helps eliminate toxins and waste products from the body. Activities such as exercise and saunas can promote sweating and support skin detoxification.

5. **Lymphatic System**: The lymphatic system is a network of vessels and lymph nodes that helps remove toxins, waste, and other unwanted substances from the body's tissues. Exercise, massage, and dry brushing can help support lymphatic drainage and detoxification.

Consequences of Toxin Accumulation

When the body's natural detoxification mechanisms become overwhelmed or compromised, toxins can accumulate, leading to various health problems.

1. **Inflammation**: Toxins can trigger inflammation in the body, which is linked to chronic diseases such as heart disease, diabetes, and autoimmune conditions.

2. **Oxidative Stress**: Toxins can generate reactive oxygen species (ROS) in the body, leading to oxidative stress. Oxidative stress damages cells, proteins, and DNA and is implicated in aging and the development of diseases such as cancer.

3. **Impaired Organ Function**: Toxins can impair the function of detoxification organs such as the liver and kidneys, leading to decreased detoxification capacity and potential health problems.

4. **Weakened Immune System**: Toxin accumulation can weaken the immune system, making the body more susceptible to infections and illnesses.

5. **Fatigue and Low Energy**: Toxins can interfere with energy production in the body, leading to fatigue, low energy levels, and feelings of sluggishness.

Supporting Detoxification for Health

Supporting the body's natural detoxification processes is essential for maintaining optimal health and well-being. Several lifestyle practices and dietary strategies can promote detoxification and support overall health.

1. **Healthy Diet**: Consuming a diet rich in whole, nutrient-dense foods such as fruits, vegetables, whole grains, lean proteins,

and healthy fats provides essential nutrients that support detoxification pathways and overall health.

2. **Hydration**: Adequate hydration supports kidney function and promotes the elimination of toxins through urine. Drinking plenty of water and herbal teas helps flush out toxins from the body.

3. **Regular Exercise**: Exercise promotes sweating, which helps eliminate toxins through the skin. Additionally, physical activity supports overall health and enhances circulation, which aids in detoxification.

4. **Stress Management**: Chronic stress can impair detoxification pathways and contribute to toxin accumulation in the body. Practices such as meditation, yoga, deep breathing exercises, and mindfulness can help reduce stress and support detoxification.

5. **Limit Exposure to Toxins**: Minimizing exposure to environmental toxins by using natural cleaning products, eating organic foods, filtering drinking water, and avoiding processed foods and artificial additives can reduce the body's toxic burden.

6. **Supportive Supplements**: Certain supplements, such as antioxidants (e.g., vitamin C, vitamin E, selenium), liver-supporting herbs (e.g., milk thistle, dandelion root), and

glutathione precursors (e.g., N-acetyl cysteine), can support detoxification pathways and enhance overall health.

Conclusion

Understanding the importance of detoxification for health involves recognizing the body's natural detoxification mechanisms, the consequences of toxin accumulation, and strategies for supporting detoxification. By adopting a healthy lifestyle, including a balanced diet, regular exercise, stress management, and minimizing exposure to toxins, individuals can promote optimal detoxification and support overall health and well-being.

CHAPTER THREE

Dr. Barbara's Philosophy on Body Detoxification

Dr. Barbara, a renowned expert in holistic health and wellness, advocates for a comprehensive approach to body detoxification that encompasses the mind, body, and spirit. Grounded in principles of naturopathic medicine and functional medicine, Dr. Barbara's philosophy emphasizes the importance of supporting the body's natural detoxification processes while addressing underlying imbalances that contribute to toxin accumulation and poor health. Central to her approach are personalized dietary and lifestyle interventions, as well as holistic modalities that promote detoxification, vitality, and overall well-being.

Holistic Approach to Detoxification

Dr. Barbara's philosophy on body detoxification centers on the understanding that detoxification is a natural, ongoing process that involves multiple systems within the body. Rather than viewing detoxification as a one-time event or quick fix, she emphasizes the importance of nurturing the body's innate ability to eliminate toxins while addressing underlying factors that may hinder this process. Dr. Barbara recognizes that detoxification is not solely physical but also involves emotional and spiritual aspects of health.

Personalized Dietary Interventions

Dr. Barbara believes that diet plays a crucial role in supporting detoxification and overall health. She advocates for a whole foods-based approach that emphasizes nutrient-dense foods rich in antioxidants, vitamins, minerals, and fiber. However, Dr. Barbara acknowledges that individual nutritional needs vary, and there is no one-size-fits-all approach to detoxification. She works closely with her clients to develop personalized dietary plans tailored to their unique health goals, preferences, and biochemical individuality.

Emphasis on Liver Support

As the primary organ responsible for detoxification, the liver plays a central role in Dr. Barbara's approach to body detoxification. She emphasizes the importance of supporting liver function through dietary interventions, targeted supplementation, and lifestyle modifications. Dr. Barbara recommends incorporating liver-supportive foods such as cruciferous vegetables, leafy greens, garlic, turmeric, and dandelion root into the diet. Additionally, she may recommend specific herbs and supplements known to enhance liver detoxification pathways, such as milk thistle, N-acetyl cysteine (NAC), and glutathione.

Mind-Body-Spirit Connection

Dr. Barbara recognizes the interconnectedness of the mind, body, and spirit in achieving optimal health and detoxification. She encourages her clients to cultivate mindfulness, stress management techniques, and practices that promote emotional well-being. Dr. Barbara believes that unresolved emotional issues and chronic stress can impact detoxification pathways and overall health. Therefore, she integrates modalities such as meditation, breathwork, yoga, and counseling into her holistic approach to detoxification.

Education and Empowerment

Central to Dr. Barbara's philosophy is the empowerment of her clients through education and self-care practices. She believes in equipping individuals with the knowledge and tools they need to take an active role in their health and well-being. Dr. Barbara educates her clients about the importance of detoxification, the role of nutrition and lifestyle factors, and how to make informed choices that support their health goals. By empowering her clients to make sustainable changes, Dr. Barbara aims to facilitate long-term health and vitality.

Conclusion

Dr. Barbara's philosophy on body detoxification reflects a holistic approach that considers the interconnectedness of the mind, body, and spirit. Grounded in principles of naturopathic and functional medicine, her approach emphasizes personalized dietary interventions, liver support, and mind-body practices to promote detoxification and overall well-being. By empowering her clients through education and self-care, Dr. Barbara strives to facilitate lasting health transformation and vitality.

CHAPTER FOUR

The Science Behind Detoxification: How It Works

Detoxification is a fundamental process in the human body that involves the neutralization and elimination of toxins and waste products. This intricate process is orchestrated by various organs, enzymes, and pathways, working together to maintain internal balance and support overall health. Understanding the science behind detoxification involves exploring the mechanisms by which toxins are processed, transformed, and excreted, as well as the role of key organs and biochemical pathways in this vital physiological process.

1. Liver Detoxification Pathways

The liver is the primary organ responsible for detoxification in the body. It employs a series of enzymatic reactions to metabolize and neutralize toxins, making them less harmful and easier to eliminate. There are two main phases of liver detoxification:

- **Phase I (Functionalization)**: During this phase, enzymes such as cytochrome P450 enzymes catalyze reactions that convert fat-soluble toxins into intermediate metabolites. This process often involves oxidation, reduction, or hydrolysis reactions, rendering the toxins more reactive and water-soluble.

- **Phase II (Conjugation)**: In this phase, the intermediate metabolites produced in Phase I are further processed through conjugation reactions, where they are combined with molecules such as glutathione, amino acids, or sulfate groups. This conjugation process makes the toxins more water-soluble and facilitates their excretion from the body via urine or bile.

2. Kidney Filtration and Excretion

The kidneys play a crucial role in detoxification by filtering waste products and toxins from the blood and excreting them in the form of urine. The glomeruli, tiny clusters of blood vessels within the kidneys, filter the blood, allowing water, electrolytes, and waste products to pass through. Subsequently, the filtered waste products, including toxins and metabolic byproducts, are concentrated in the urine and eliminated from the body.

3. Intestinal Elimination

The gastrointestinal tract also contributes to detoxification through the elimination of waste products and toxins via feces. Bile, produced by the liver and stored in the gallbladder, contains toxins and waste products that have been processed by the liver. Bile is released into the small intestine, where it emulsifies fats and facilitates the absorption of nutrients. Additionally, fiber-rich foods help bind toxins in the gut, preventing their reabsorption, and promoting their excretion through feces.

4. Skin and Lung Detoxification

While the liver, kidneys, and intestines are the primary organs involved in detoxification, the skin and lungs also play supportive roles. The skin eliminates toxins through sweating, a process that helps regulate body temperature and remove metabolic waste products. Sweating during physical activity, saunas, or hot baths can promote skin detoxification. Additionally, the lungs excrete volatile toxins and waste products through exhalation, contributing to the overall detoxification process.

5. Antioxidant Defense System

Detoxification is closely linked to the body's antioxidant defense system, which helps protect cells from oxidative damage caused by free radicals and reactive oxygen species (ROS). Antioxidants such as vitamins C and E, glutathione, and enzymes like superoxide dismutase (SOD) neutralize free radicals and support cellular health. By reducing oxidative stress, antioxidants play a critical role in detoxification and overall health.

Conclusion

Detoxification is a complex physiological process involving multiple organs, enzymes, and pathways working together to eliminate toxins and maintain internal balance. The liver, kidneys, intestines, skin, and lungs play key roles in detoxification, supported by the body's antioxidant defense system.

Understanding the science behind detoxification provides insights into how lifestyle factors, such as diet, hydration, exercise, and stress management, can influence this essential process and support overall health and well-being.

CHAPTER FIVE

Essential Foods for Supporting Detoxification

A well-balanced diet rich in nutrient-dense foods can support the body's natural detoxification processes, enhance liver function, and promote overall health and well-being. Incorporating specific foods that contain detoxifying properties can help eliminate toxins, reduce inflammation, and support organ function. Below are essential foods that can support detoxification:

1. Cruciferous Vegetables

Cruciferous vegetables such as broccoli, cabbage, cauliflower, Brussels sprouts, and kale are rich in compounds called glucosinolates, which are known for their potent detoxification properties. These compounds are broken down into bioactive substances like sulforaphane, which supports liver detoxification enzymes and enhances the elimination of toxins from the body.

2. Leafy Greens

Leafy greens such as spinach, kale, Swiss chard, and collard greens are nutritional powerhouses packed with vitamins, minerals, and antioxidants. They contain chlorophyll, a natural pigment that supports detoxification by binding to toxins and aiding in their elimination. Leafy greens are also rich in fiber, which promotes bowel regularity and helps remove waste products from the body.

3. Berries

Berries such as blueberries, strawberries, raspberries, and blackberries are loaded with antioxidants, including vitamin C, flavonoids, and polyphenols, which help neutralize free radicals and reduce oxidative stress. These antioxidants support cellular health and contribute to detoxification by protecting cells from damage caused by toxins and metabolic byproducts.

4. Garlic and Onions

Garlic and onions are members of the allium family and are known for their potent detoxification properties. They contain sulfur-containing compounds such as allicin and sulfoxides, which support liver detoxification enzymes and enhance the elimination of toxins from the body. Additionally, garlic and onions have antibacterial and antiviral properties, supporting immune function and overall health.

5. Turmeric

Turmeric, a spice commonly used in Indian cuisine, contains a bioactive compound called curcumin, which has powerful anti-inflammatory and antioxidant properties. Curcumin supports liver detoxification pathways, reduces inflammation, and protects against oxidative damage. Incorporating turmeric into dishes or consuming it as a supplement can support detoxification and overall health.

6. Ginger

Ginger is well-known for its anti-inflammatory and digestive properties. It contains bioactive compounds such as gingerol and shogaol, which have been shown to support liver function and promote detoxification. Ginger also aids in digestion, reduces bloating, and supports gastrointestinal health, making it a valuable addition to a detoxifying diet.

7. Lemon and Citrus Fruits

Lemons and other citrus fruits such as oranges, grapefruits, and limes are rich in vitamin C, a powerful antioxidant that supports detoxification and immune function. Drinking warm lemon water in the morning can stimulate digestion, support liver function, and promote hydration, making it an excellent addition to a detoxifying regimen.

8. Green Tea

Green tea contains catechins, powerful antioxidants that support liver function and enhance detoxification. Drinking green tea regularly can help boost metabolism, improve digestion, and reduce inflammation. Green tea also contains L-theanine, an amino acid that promotes relaxation and mental clarity, making it a beneficial beverage for overall health and well-being.

Conclusion

Incorporating these essential foods into your diet can support the body's natural detoxification processes, enhance liver function, and promote overall health and well-being. By focusing on nutrient-dense whole foods rich in antioxidants, vitamins, minerals, and fiber, you can support your body's ability to eliminate toxins and maintain optimal health. Additionally, staying hydrated, engaging in regular physical activity, managing stress, and avoiding exposure to environmental toxins are important factors in supporting detoxification and overall wellness.

CHAPTER SIX

Creating a meal plan

Creating a meal plan for a detox involves incorporating nutrient-dense foods while avoiding processed foods, refined sugars, caffeine, alcohol, and potential allergens. Here's a sample 7-day detox meal plan along with recipes for each day:

Day 1:

Breakfast: Green Smoothie

- 1 cup spinach
- 1/2 cup kale
- 1/2 banana
- 1/2 cup pineapple
- 1/2 cup almond milk
- 1 tablespoon chia seeds

Lunch: Quinoa Salad

- 1 cup cooked quinoa
- 1/2 cup cherry tomatoes, halved
- 1/2 cucumber, diced
- 1/4 cup diced red onion

- 1/4 cup chopped fresh parsley

- Juice of 1 lemon

- 2 tablespoons extra virgin olive oil

- Salt and pepper to taste

Dinner: Baked Salmon with Steamed Broccoli

- 4 oz salmon fillet

- 1 tablespoon olive oil

- 1 teaspoon lemon zest

- 1 clove garlic, minced

- Salt and pepper to taste

- 1 cup steamed broccoli

Day 2:

Breakfast: Chia Seed Pudding

- 2 tablespoons chia seeds

- 1/2 cup almond milk

- 1/2 teaspoon vanilla extract

- 1/2 tablespoon maple syrup

- Fresh berries for topping

Lunch: Lentil Vegetable Soup

- 1 cup cooked lentils

- 2 cups vegetable broth

- 1 carrot, diced

- 1 celery stalk, diced

- 1/2 onion, diced

- 1 garlic clove, minced

- 1/2 teaspoon ground cumin

- Salt and pepper to taste

Dinner: Grilled Chicken with Roasted Sweet Potatoes and Asparagus

- 4 oz grilled chicken breast

- 1 medium sweet potato, cubed and roasted

- 1 cup asparagus spears, roasted with olive oil, salt, and pepper

Day 3:

Breakfast: Overnight Oats

- 1/2 cup rolled oats

- 1/2 cup almond milk

- 1 tablespoon maple syrup

- 1/2 teaspoon cinnamon

- Sliced banana and walnuts for topping

Lunch: Mixed Green Salad with Avocado

- Mixed greens

- Cherry tomatoes

- Cucumber slices

- Avocado slices

- Balsamic vinaigrette dressing

Dinner: Stir-Fried Tofu with Vegetables

- 4 oz tofu, cubed

- Mixed stir-fry vegetables (bell peppers, broccoli, carrots)

- 1 tablespoon soy sauce

- 1 teaspoon sesame oil

- 1 clove garlic, minced

- Cooked brown rice

Day 4:

Breakfast: Berry Smoothie Bowl

- 1 cup mixed berries (strawberries, blueberries, raspberries)

- 1/2 banana

- 1/2 cup almond milk

- Toppings: sliced almonds, shredded coconut, chia seeds

Lunch: Quinoa and Black Bean Salad

- 1 cup cooked quinoa

- 1/2 cup black beans, rinsed and drained

- Diced bell peppers, red onion, cilantro

- Lime vinaigrette dressing

Dinner: Grilled Shrimp with Zucchini Noodles

- 4 oz grilled shrimp

- Zucchini noodles sautéed with garlic and olive oil

- Cherry tomatoes

Day 5:

Breakfast: Greek Yogurt Parfait

- Plain Greek yogurt

- Mixed berries

- Granola

- Drizzle of honey

Lunch: Chickpea Salad

- 1 cup cooked chickpeas

- Diced cucumber, tomato, red onion

- Chopped parsley

- Lemon-tahini dressing

Dinner: Baked Cod with Roasted Vegetables

- 4 oz cod fillet

- Mixed roasted vegetables (bell peppers, zucchini, eggplant) tossed with olive oil, garlic, and herbs

Day 6:

Breakfast: Almond Butter Banana Toast

- Whole grain toast

- Almond butter

- Sliced banana

- Sprinkle of cinnamon

Lunch: Spinach and Strawberry Salad

- Baby spinach

- Sliced strawberries

- Toasted almonds

- Feta cheese

- Balsamic vinaigrette dressing

Dinner: Vegetable Stir-Fry with Brown Rice

- Mixed stir-fry vegetables (broccoli, bell peppers, snap peas)

- Tofu or tempeh

- Soy-ginger sauce

- Served over brown rice

Day 7:

Breakfast: Vegetable Omelette

- Eggs

- Diced bell peppers, onions, spinach

- Feta cheese

- Fresh herbs

Lunch: Quinoa and Vegetable Soup

- Vegetable broth

- Cooked quinoa

- Mixed vegetables (carrots, celery, kale)

- Garlic, onion, herbs

- Squeeze of lemon juice

Dinner: Lentil Stew with Sautéed Greens

- Lentils cooked with diced tomatoes, garlic, onion, and spices

- Sautéed greens (kale, Swiss chard) with garlic and lemon juice

Conclusion:

This sample 7-day detox meal plan provides a variety of nutritious and flavorful recipes to support your detoxification journey. Remember to stay hydrated throughout the day by drinking plenty of water and herbal teas. Additionally, listen to your body's hunger and fullness cues, and adjust portion sizes as needed. Feel free to modify these recipes based on your dietary preferences and consult with a healthcare professional before making significant changes to your diet, especially if you have any underlying health conditions.

CHAPTER SEVEN

Incorporating detoxifying practices into your routine

Incorporating detoxifying practices into your routine can support your body's natural detoxification processes, enhance overall health, and promote a sense of well-being. These practices involve lifestyle habits and self-care rituals that help eliminate toxins, reduce stress, and support optimal functioning of organs such as the liver, kidneys, and lymphatic system. Here are some effective ways to incorporate detoxifying practices into your daily routine:

1. Hydration:

Start your day with a glass of warm water with lemon to support hydration and kickstart your metabolism. Throughout the day, aim to drink plenty of water to help flush out toxins from your system. Herbal teas, such as dandelion root tea or green tea, can also support detoxification and provide additional hydration.

2. Clean Eating:

Focus on incorporating whole, nutrient-dense foods into your diet, such as fruits, vegetables, whole grains, lean proteins, and healthy fats. Avoid processed foods, refined sugars, artificial additives, and trans fats, which can contribute to toxin buildup in the body. Consider incorporating detoxifying foods and herbs into your meals, such as garlic, onions, cruciferous vegetables, ginger, turmeric, and leafy greens.

3. Mindful Eating:

Practice mindful eating by paying attention to your hunger and fullness cues, chewing your food thoroughly, and savoring each bite. Avoid distractions such as screens or multitasking while eating, as this can lead to overeating and poor digestion. Eating mindfully can help improve digestion, nutrient absorption, and overall satisfaction with your meals.

4. Regular Exercise:

Incorporate regular physical activity into your routine to support circulation, lymphatic drainage, and overall detoxification. Choose activities that you enjoy, such as walking, jogging, swimming, yoga, or dancing, and aim for at least 30 minutes of moderate-intensity exercise most days of the week. Sweating during exercise helps eliminate toxins through the skin and promotes overall well-being.

5. Deep Breathing and Relaxation Techniques:

Practice deep breathing exercises, meditation, or mindfulness techniques to reduce stress and promote relaxation. Stress can impair detoxification pathways and contribute to toxin buildup in the body, so it's essential to incorporate stress management practices into your routine. Try taking a few minutes each day to focus on your breath, engage in guided meditation, or practice progressive muscle relaxation to calm the mind and body.

6. Dry Brushing:

Consider incorporating dry brushing into your skincare routine to promote lymphatic drainage and exfoliation. Using a natural bristle brush, gently brush your skin in upward strokes towards the heart before showering. Dry brushing helps stimulate circulation, remove dead skin cells, and support the body's natural detoxification process through the lymphatic system.

7. Sauna or Steam Therapy:

If available, consider incorporating sauna or steam therapy into your routine to promote sweating and detoxification. Spending time in a sauna or steam room helps open up pores, increase circulation, and eliminate toxins through the skin. Be sure to stay hydrated before, during, and after sauna sessions to support hydration and replenish electrolytes lost through sweating.

8. Adequate Sleep:

Prioritize getting enough sleep each night to support detoxification, hormone balance, and overall health. Aim for 7-9 hours of quality sleep per night, and establish a relaxing bedtime routine to signal to your body that it's time to wind down. Create a sleep-friendly environment by keeping your bedroom dark, quiet, and cool, and avoid screens and stimulating activities before bedtime.

Incorporating these detoxifying practices into your daily routine can support your body's natural detoxification processes, enhance overall health, and promote a sense of well-being. Experiment with different practices to find what works best for you, and make self-care a priority in your daily life.

CHAPTER EIGHT

Hydration and supplements

Hydration and supplements play essential roles in supporting optimal detoxification results by promoting the elimination of toxins, replenishing essential nutrients, and supporting the overall health of detoxification organs. Here's how to optimize hydration and supplement intake for effective detoxification:

Hydration:

1. **Water:** Adequate hydration is crucial for supporting detoxification processes. Drink plenty of water throughout the day to help flush out toxins from your system and support kidney function. Aim for at least 8-10 glasses of water daily, or more if you're exercising or in a hot environment.

2. **Herbal Teas:** Incorporate herbal teas such as dandelion root, green tea, ginger tea, or milk thistle tea into your routine. These teas not only provide hydration but also contain compounds that support liver function and detoxification.

3. **Electrolyte Balance:** Ensure you maintain electrolyte balance by consuming foods rich in potassium, magnesium, and sodium. Electrolytes help regulate fluid balance, muscle function, and nerve function. Include foods like bananas, leafy greens, nuts, seeds, and coconut water in your diet.

Supplements:

1. **Multivitamin and Mineral:** A high-quality multivitamin and mineral supplement can help fill in nutritional gaps and provide essential nutrients needed for detoxification. Look for a supplement that contains a wide range of vitamins and minerals, including vitamin C, vitamin E, B vitamins, magnesium, selenium, zinc, and chromium.

2. **Omega-3 Fatty Acids:** Omega-3 fatty acids, found in fish oil or algae supplements, have anti-inflammatory properties and support overall health. They can help reduce inflammation and support detoxification pathways in the body. Consider taking a fish oil or algae supplement daily to support your detox efforts.

3. **Antioxidants:** Antioxidants such as vitamin C, vitamin E, selenium, and glutathione help neutralize free radicals and reduce oxidative stress in the body. Consider supplementing with antioxidants or consuming foods rich in antioxidants, such as berries, citrus fruits, nuts, seeds, and dark leafy greens.

4. **Liver Support:** Certain supplements can support liver function and enhance detoxification processes. Milk thistle, N-acetyl cysteine (NAC), turmeric, dandelion root, and alpha-lipoic acid are examples of supplements that support liver health and detoxification. Consult with a healthcare

professional before adding new supplements to your regimen, especially if you have any underlying health conditions or are taking medications.

5. **Probiotics:** Probiotics are beneficial bacteria that support gut health and digestion. Maintaining a healthy balance of gut bacteria is essential for proper detoxification and elimination of toxins. Consider taking a high-quality probiotic supplement to support gut health during your detoxification process.

6. **Digestive Enzymes:** Digestive enzymes help break down food and facilitate nutrient absorption. Supplementing with digestive enzymes can support digestion and nutrient absorption, which is essential for overall health and detoxification. Look for a broad-spectrum digestive enzyme supplement that contains proteases, lipases, and amylases.

7. **Hydrolyzed Collagen:** Collagen is the most abundant protein in the body and is essential for skin, joint, and gut health. Supplementing with hydrolyzed collagen can support detoxification by promoting gut health and supporting connective tissue repair. Consider adding a collagen supplement to your routine to support overall health during detoxification.

Conclusion:

Hydration and supplementation are essential components of an effective detoxification regimen. By staying properly hydrated and incorporating targeted supplements into your routine, you can support the body's natural detoxification processes, promote optimal health, and enhance the results of your detox efforts. However, it's essential to consult with a healthcare professional before starting any new supplement regimen, especially if you have any underlying health conditions or are taking medications. They can help you determine the most appropriate supplements for your individual needs and ensure they won't interact with any medications you may be taking.

CHAPTER NINE

detox symptoms and challenges

Addressing detox symptoms and challenges is an important aspect of any detoxification program. Detox symptoms can vary widely from person to person and may include fatigue, headaches, digestive issues, skin breakouts, mood swings, and flu-like symptoms. These symptoms often occur as the body adjusts to the changes in diet, lifestyle, and toxin release. Here's how to address detox symptoms and challenges effectively:

1. Gradual Transition:

- Ease into your detox program gradually to minimize detox symptoms. Start by eliminating processed foods, caffeine, alcohol, and sugar from your diet before embarking on a more restrictive detox plan.

- Gradually increase your intake of detoxifying foods and beverages while gradually reducing your intake of potential toxins.

2. Stay Hydrated:

- Drink plenty of water and herbal teas throughout the day to support hydration and help flush out toxins from your system.

- Proper hydration can help alleviate detox symptoms such as headaches, fatigue, and digestive issues.

3. Support Liver Health:

- Support liver function with liver-supportive foods and supplements such as milk thistle, dandelion root, turmeric, and N-acetyl cysteine (NAC).

- Liver-supportive herbs and nutrients can help enhance detoxification pathways and alleviate detox symptoms.

4. Supportive Supplements:

- Consider taking supplements that support detoxification and reduce detox symptoms, such as glutathione, vitamin C, magnesium, and B vitamins.

- Consult with a healthcare professional before starting any new supplement regimen to ensure they are safe and appropriate for your individual needs.

5. Gentle Exercise:

- Engage in gentle exercise such as walking, yoga, or swimming to support circulation, lymphatic drainage, and toxin elimination.

- Exercise can help alleviate detox symptoms, improve mood, and enhance overall well-being.

6. Stress Management:

- Practice stress management techniques such as deep breathing, meditation, yoga, or tai chi to reduce stress and support detoxification.

- Chronic stress can impair detoxification pathways and exacerbate detox symptoms, so it's essential to prioritize stress reduction during your detox program.

7. Rest and Relaxation:

- Get plenty of rest and prioritize relaxation during your detox program. Aim for 7-9 hours of quality sleep per night to support detoxification and overall health.

- Take time to rest and recharge, especially if you're experiencing fatigue or other detox symptoms.

8. Listen to Your Body:

- Pay attention to your body's signals and listen to what it needs during your detox program.

- If you're experiencing severe or prolonged detox symptoms, consider modifying your detox plan or seeking guidance from a healthcare professional.

9. Address Emotional Release:

- Detoxification can sometimes trigger emotional release as stored toxins are released from the body. Practice self-care and seek support from friends, family, or a counselor if needed.

- Journaling, meditation, and mindfulness practices can help process emotions and support emotional well-being during detoxification.

10. Seek Professional Guidance:

- If you're experiencing significant or persistent detox symptoms, consider seeking guidance from a healthcare professional, such as a naturopathic doctor or functional medicine practitioner.

- A healthcare professional can help you navigate detox symptoms, tailor a detox program to your individual needs, and address any underlying health issues that may be contributing to detox challenges.

By addressing detox symptoms and challenges effectively, you can support your body's natural detoxification processes, minimize discomfort, and promote overall health and well-being. Remember to listen to your body, practice self-care, and seek professional guidance if needed to ensure a safe and effective detoxification experience.

CHAPTER TEN

Long-term health maintenance

Long-term health maintenance is essential for sustaining the benefits of a detox program and supporting overall health and well-being. After completing a detox, it's important to implement post-detox guidelines and lifestyle changes to continue supporting your body's natural detoxification processes and maintain optimal health. Here are some post-detox guidelines and lifestyle changes to consider:

1. Balanced Diet:

- Continue to prioritize a balanced diet rich in whole, nutrient-dense foods such as fruits, vegetables, whole grains, lean proteins, and healthy fats.

- Aim to include a variety of colorful fruits and vegetables in your meals to provide a wide range of vitamins, minerals, antioxidants, and phytonutrients.

2. Hydration:

- Maintain adequate hydration by drinking plenty of water throughout the day. Aim for at least 8-10 glasses of water daily, or more if you're exercising or in a hot environment.

- Continue to incorporate herbal teas and hydrating beverages into your routine to support hydration and detoxification.

3. Regular Exercise:

- Make regular physical activity a priority in your routine to support circulation, lymphatic drainage, and overall health.

- Choose activities that you enjoy and aim for at least 30 minutes of moderate-intensity exercise most days of the week.

4. Stress Management:

- Continue to practice stress management techniques such as deep breathing, meditation, yoga, or tai chi to reduce stress and promote relaxation.

- Prioritize self-care activities that help you unwind and recharge, such as spending time in nature, engaging in hobbies, or connecting with loved ones.

5. Sleep Hygiene:

- Maintain healthy sleep habits by prioritizing regular sleep schedules and creating a relaxing bedtime routine.

- Aim for 7-9 hours of quality sleep per night to support detoxification, hormone balance, and overall health.

6. Limit Exposure to Toxins:

- Minimize exposure to environmental toxins by choosing natural and organic products whenever possible.

- Avoid processed foods, artificial additives, pesticides, and pollutants, and opt for whole, organic foods whenever possible.

7. Mindful Eating:

- Continue to practice mindful eating by paying attention to your hunger and fullness cues, chewing your food thoroughly, and savoring each bite.

- Avoid overeating, emotional eating, and mindless snacking, and focus on nourishing your body with nutrient-dense foods.

8. Regular Detox Support:

- Consider incorporating regular detox support practices into your routine, such as occasional juice cleanses, detoxifying baths, or sauna sessions.

- These practices can help support your body's natural detoxification processes and promote overall health and well-being.

9. Routine Health Screenings:

- Schedule routine health screenings and check-ups with your healthcare provider to monitor your health status and address any underlying health issues.

- Regular screenings can help detect potential health problems early and facilitate timely intervention and treatment.

10. Continuous Learning and Adaptation:

- Stay informed about the latest research and recommendations related to nutrition, lifestyle, and wellness.

- Remain open to making adjustments to your diet, lifestyle, and self-care practices as needed to support your evolving health goals and needs.

By incorporating these post-detox guidelines and lifestyle changes into your routine, you can continue to support your body's natural detoxification processes, maintain optimal health, and enjoy long-term well-being. Remember that consistency and commitment to healthy habits are key to achieving sustainable health outcomes over time.

BONUS: SOME HERBAL AND HOLISTIC APPROACHES TO KNOW

Steam Baths:

Definition: Steam baths, also known as steam rooms or steam saunas, are enclosed spaces where hot, humid air is generated by boiling water and released into the room. Steam baths are used for relaxation, detoxification, and promoting overall health and well-being.

Ingredients: Steam baths require water and a heat source, typically a steam generator or boiler, to produce steam. The steam itself is the active ingredient in steam baths, providing heat and humidity to the body.

How to Prepare: Preparing for a steam bath involves selecting a suitable steam room or facility and ensuring that it's properly heated and ventilated. It's essential to hydrate adequately before and after a steam bath to prevent dehydration and to listen to your body's cues to avoid overheating.

Dosage: The duration and frequency of steam bath sessions can vary depending on individual preferences and tolerance to heat. A typical steam bath session may last 10 to 20 minutes, although some people may prefer shorter or longer sessions.

How to Use: To use a steam bath, enter the steam room and sit or lie comfortably, allowing the hot, humid air to envelop your body. It's important to breathe deeply and relax during the session, allowing the steam to penetrate the skin and promote sweating and detoxification. After the designated time, exit the steam room, cool down gradually, and rehydrate with water or electrolyte-rich beverages.

Side Effects: Steam baths are generally safe for most people when used appropriately, but they can pose risks if not practiced correctly. Potential side effects of steam baths may include dehydration, heat exhaustion, heatstroke, dizziness, fainting, and exacerbation of certain medical conditions (such as cardiovascular disease or low blood pressure). It's important to stay hydrated, limit steam bath sessions to a safe duration, and avoid excessive heat exposure if pregnant, breastfeeding, or if you have certain health conditions. Individuals with underlying health concerns should consult with a healthcare provider before starting steam bath therapy to ensure it's safe and appropriate for them.

Sugar Detox:

Definition: A sugar detox is a dietary approach aimed at reducing or eliminating added sugars from the diet for a specified period. It's designed to break dependence on sugar, reset taste buds, improve metabolic health, and reduce cravings for sweet foods.

Ingredients: A sugar detox involves eliminating or minimizing foods and beverages that contain added sugars, such as sugary snacks, desserts, sweetened beverages, processed foods, and condiments with added sugars. Instead, it emphasizes whole, unprocessed foods such as fruits, vegetables, lean proteins, whole grains, nuts, seeds, and healthy fats.

How to Prepare: Preparing for a sugar detox involves cleaning out your pantry and refrigerator of sugary foods and stocking up on nutritious, whole foods. It's essential to read food labels carefully to identify hidden sources of added sugars and to plan meals and snacks that are free from added sugars.

Dosage: The duration of a sugar detox can vary depending on individual goals and preferences. Some people may choose to do a short-term sugar detox lasting a few days to a week, while others may opt for a longer-term approach lasting several weeks or more. It's important to set realistic goals and listen to your body's cues during the detox process.

How to Use: During a sugar detox, focus on eating whole, nutrient-dense foods that are naturally low in sugar and high in fiber, protein, and healthy fats. This may include plenty of fruits and vegetables, lean proteins such as poultry, fish, tofu, and legumes, whole grains such as quinoa and brown rice, nuts and seeds, and healthy fats such as avocados and olive oil. Be mindful of your sugar intake from natural sources such as fruits and limit added sugars from processed foods and beverages.

Side Effects: A sugar detox may initially cause side effects such as cravings, mood swings, headaches, fatigue, and irritability as the body adjusts to lower sugar intake. These symptoms are usually temporary and subside with time. It's important to stay hydrated, eat balanced meals, and get plenty of sleep during the detox process to support overall well-being. If you have specific health concerns or medical conditions, consult with a healthcare provider or registered dietitian before starting a sugar detox to ensure it's safe and appropriate for you.

Superfood Detox:

Definition: A superfood detox is a dietary approach that focuses on incorporating nutrient-dense superfoods into the diet to support detoxification, boost energy levels, and promote overall health and well-being. Superfoods are foods that are exceptionally high in vitamins, minerals, antioxidants, and other beneficial compounds.

Ingredients: A superfood detox emphasizes consuming a variety of superfoods such as leafy greens (like kale, spinach, and Swiss chard), berries (such as blueberries, strawberries, and raspberries), cruciferous vegetables (like broccoli, cauliflower, and Brussels sprouts), nuts and seeds (such as almonds, chia seeds, and flaxseeds), fatty fish (such as salmon and sardines), whole grains (like quinoa and barley), and herbs and spices (such as turmeric, ginger, and garlic).

How to Prepare: Preparing for a superfood detox involves incorporating a wide range of nutrient-dense superfoods into your meals and snacks. It's essential to plan meals that include a variety of colors, textures, and flavors to ensure a diverse intake of nutrients.

Dosage: There isn't a specific dosage for a superfood detox, as it depends on individual preferences, dietary needs, and health goals. Aim to include a variety of superfoods in your diet regularly to maximize nutrient intake and support overall health and well-being.

How to Use: To incorporate superfoods into your diet, focus on eating a balanced diet that includes a variety of nutrient-dense foods from all food groups. Include superfoods in your meals and snacks in creative ways, such as adding berries to smoothies, topping salads with nuts and seeds, incorporating leafy greens into soups and stir-fries, and seasoning dishes with herbs and spices.

Side Effects: A superfood detox is generally safe for most people when part of a balanced diet and healthy lifestyle. However, consuming large quantities of certain superfoods or relying solely on superfoods for nutrition may lead to imbalances or nutrient deficiencies. It's essential to eat a varied diet that includes a wide range of nutrient-dense foods to ensure adequate intake of all essential nutrients. If you have specific health concerns or medical conditions, consult with a healthcare provider or registered dietitian before starting a superfood detox to ensure it's safe and appropriate for you.

Sweating:

Definition: Sweating is the body's natural process of producing sweat, a clear fluid secreted by sweat glands in response to heat, physical exertion, stress, or emotional stimuli. Sweating plays a crucial role in regulating body temperature, removing toxins and metabolic waste products, and maintaining hydration and electrolyte balance.

Ingredients: Sweating requires no specific ingredients but is influenced by factors such as environmental temperature, physical activity level, hydration status, and individual metabolic rate. The primary component of sweat is water, along with small amounts of electrolytes, urea, ammonia, and other waste products.

How to Prepare: Preparing for sweating involves creating conditions that promote perspiration, such as engaging in physical activity, spending time in a hot environment (such as a sauna or steam room), or wearing appropriate clothing for exercise or outdoor activities.

Dosage: The amount and intensity of sweating can vary depending on factors such as environmental conditions, physical activity level, and individual physiology. It's essential to listen to your body's cues and stay hydrated during sweating to prevent dehydration and electrolyte imbalances.

How to Use: To promote sweating, engage in activities that raise body temperature and induce perspiration, such as exercise, hot baths or showers, sauna sessions, steam baths, or participating in hot yoga or other heated fitness classes. Make sure to stay hydrated by drinking water or electrolyte-rich beverages before, during, and after sweating to replace lost fluids and minerals.

Side Effects: Sweating is generally considered a healthy and natural bodily function, but excessive sweating (hyperhidrosis) or sweating in certain circumstances (such as heatstroke) can lead to dehydration, electrolyte imbalances, heat-related illness, and skin irritation. It's essential to practice proper hydration and listen to your body's signals to prevent overheating and dehydration during sweating. If you experience persistent or excessive sweating, consult with a healthcare provider to rule out underlying medical conditions or seek appropriate treatment.

TCM (Traditional Chinese Medicine) Detox:

Definition: Traditional Chinese Medicine (TCM) detox is a holistic approach to cleansing and detoxification based on principles of balance and harmony within the body. It involves using various TCM modalities such as acupuncture, herbal medicine, dietary therapy, cupping, and qigong to support the body's natural detoxification processes and restore optimal health and vitality.

Ingredients: TCM detox utilizes a combination of natural ingredients such as medicinal herbs, botanical extracts, acupuncture needles, dietary recommendations, and lifestyle modifications to promote detoxification and balance within the body. Specific herbs and formulas may be prescribed based on individual constitution, health concerns, and patterns of disharmony according to TCM principles.

How to Prepare: Preparing for a TCM detox involves consulting with a qualified TCM practitioner to assess your health status, identify imbalances or blockages within the body, and develop a personalized treatment plan tailored to your specific needs and goals. This may involve a combination of acupuncture sessions, herbal medicine prescriptions, dietary recommendations, and lifestyle modifications.

Dosage: The duration and frequency of TCM detox treatments can vary depending on individual health goals, the severity of symptoms, and response to treatment. TCM detox may involve a series of acupuncture sessions, herbal medicine formulas, dietary adjustments, and lifestyle recommendations over several weeks or months to achieve optimal results.

How to Use: To undergo a TCM detox, schedule regular appointments with a qualified TCM practitioner who can provide acupuncture treatments, prescribe herbal medicine formulas, offer dietary and lifestyle guidance, and monitor your progress throughout the detoxification process. Follow your practitioner's recommendations closely and incorporate TCM principles into your daily routine to support detoxification and overall well-being.

Side Effects: TCM detox is generally safe and well-tolerated when administered by a qualified practitioner, but some individuals may experience mild side effects such as temporary soreness or bruising at acupuncture sites, digestive upset from herbal medicine formulas, or changes in energy levels or mood as the body adjusts to detoxification. It's essential to communicate openly with your TCM practitioner about any concerns or reactions you may experience during treatment and to follow their guidance for managing side effects and optimizing treatment outcomes. If you have underlying health conditions or are pregnant or breastfeeding, consult with a healthcare provider before starting a TCM detox to ensure it's safe and appropriate for you.

Turmeric Supplements:

Definition: Turmeric supplements are dietary supplements containing extracts of turmeric, a golden-yellow spice derived from the rhizomes of the Curcuma longa plant. Turmeric is well-known for its active compound, curcumin, which exhibits potent antioxidant and anti-inflammatory properties.

Ingredients: Turmeric supplements typically contain concentrated extracts of turmeric rhizomes standardized to contain specific amounts of curcumin, along with other bioactive compounds found in turmeric. Additional ingredients may include black pepper extract (piperine) to enhance the absorption of curcumin and fillers or binders used in capsule or tablet formulations.

How to Prepare: Preparing for turmeric supplement use involves selecting a high-quality product from a reputable manufacturer and following the recommended dosage instructions provided on the product packaging or as advised by a healthcare provider. It's essential to choose supplements that are standardized to contain a clinically effective dose of curcumin and free from contaminants or additives.

Dosage: The recommended dosage of turmeric supplements can vary depending on the specific formulation, concentration of curcumin, and individual health needs. Typical doses range from 500 mg to 2000 mg of turmeric extract per day, taken with meals to enhance absorption. It's important to follow the dosage instructions carefully and not exceed the recommended dose without consulting with a healthcare provider.

How to Use: Turmeric supplements are typically taken orally with water or another beverage, preferably with meals to enhance absorption. Some supplements may recommend taking them at specific times of the day or with certain foods to optimize absorption and efficacy. It's essential to take turmeric supplements consistently as part of a daily routine to maximize their potential health benefits.

Side Effects: Turmeric supplements are generally safe for most people when used as directed, but some individuals may experience side effects such as gastrointestinal upset, nausea, diarrhea, or allergic reactions. High doses of curcumin may interact with certain medications or have blood-thinning effects, so it's important to consult with a healthcare provider before using turmeric supplements, especially if you have underlying health conditions or are taking medications. Pregnant or breastfeeding women and individuals with gallbladder issues or bile duct obstruction should avoid high doses of turmeric supplements. It's also essential to choose supplements from reputable brands with third-party testing and certifications to ensure product quality and purity.

Vegetable Juices:

Definition: Vegetable juices are beverages made by extracting the liquid content from fresh vegetables, either through juicing or blending, to create a nutrient-dense and refreshing drink. Vegetable juices are rich in vitamins, minerals, antioxidants, and phytonutrients, providing numerous health benefits.

Ingredients: Vegetable juices can be made from a variety of fresh vegetables, including leafy greens (such as spinach, kale, and

Swiss chard), carrots, cucumbers, celery, beets, bell peppers, tomatoes, and root vegetables (such as ginger and turmeric). Additional ingredients may include fruits for sweetness or flavor enhancement, herbs, and spices.

How to Prepare: Preparing vegetable juices involves selecting fresh, organic vegetables and washing them thoroughly before juicing or blending. Some people prefer using a juicer to extract the liquid from vegetables, while others may use a high-speed blender to make vegetable smoothies or juices with added fiber.

Dosage: There isn't a specific dosage for vegetable juices, as it depends on individual preferences and dietary needs. Some people may choose to drink vegetable juices as part of a daily routine, while others may incorporate them into a periodic juice cleanse or detox regimen. It's essential to listen to your body's cues and consume vegetable juices in moderation as part of a balanced diet.

How to Use: To enjoy vegetable juices, simply juice or blend your favorite vegetables and fruits into a refreshing beverage. You can customize vegetable juice recipes to suit your taste preferences and nutritional goals by experimenting with different combinations of ingredients. Vegetable juices can be consumed on their own as a snack or meal replacement, or alongside other foods as part of a balanced meal.

Side Effects: Vegetable juices are generally safe for most people when consumed as part of a balanced diet, but some individuals may experience side effects such as digestive upset, gas, bloating, or changes in bowel movements, especially if they're sensitive to certain vegetables or fiber-rich foods. It's essential to start with small servings of vegetable juices and gradually increase intake to assess tolerance and prevent gastrointestinal discomfort. If you have specific health concerns or medical conditions, consult with a healthcare provider or registered dietitian before starting a vegetable juice regimen to ensure it's safe and appropriate for you.

Water Fasting:

Definition: Water fasting is a type of fasting in which individuals abstain from consuming all food and drink except water for a specified period. It's often used for religious, spiritual, or health reasons, and it's believed to promote detoxification, weight loss, and various health benefits by allowing the body to rest and reset.

Ingredients: Water fasting requires only water as the sole beverage consumed during the fasting period. It excludes all other food and drink, including juices, herbal teas, and other liquids.

How to Prepare: Preparing for a water fast involves gradually reducing food intake leading up to the fasting period to minimize potential side effects such as hunger, headaches, and fatigue. It's essential to stay hydrated by drinking plenty of water throughout the fast and to listen to your body's signals to ensure you're meeting your hydration needs.

Dosage: The duration of a water fast can vary depending on individual goals, preferences, and health status. Some people may choose to fast for short periods, such as 24 to 48 hours, while others may opt for longer fasts lasting several days or even weeks. It's important to approach water fasting cautiously and to consult with a healthcare provider before attempting an extended fast, especially if you have underlying health conditions or are taking medications.

How to Use: During a water fast, individuals abstain from consuming all food and drink except water for the designated fasting period. It's essential to stay hydrated by drinking water regularly throughout the fast and to rest as needed to conserve energy. Some people may choose to engage in light activities such as walking or gentle stretching during a water fast, while others may prefer to rest more extensively.

Side Effects: Water fasting can have various side effects, especially during the initial stages as the body adjusts to the fasting state. Common side effects may include hunger, fatigue, headaches, dizziness, lightheadedness, weakness, and difficulty concentrating. In some cases, water fasting may lead to more severe complications such as electrolyte imbalances, dehydration, nutrient deficiencies, muscle loss, and impaired immune function. It's essential to approach water fasting cautiously, to listen to your body's cues, and to discontinue the fast if you experience significant discomfort or adverse effects. If you have underlying health conditions or are pregnant, breastfeeding, or menstruating, consult with a healthcare provider before attempting a water fast to ensure it's safe and appropriate for you.

Zeolite Supplements:

Definition: Zeolite supplements are dietary supplements containing zeolites, natural minerals with unique porous structures that have been used for various purposes, including water purification, industrial applications, and as dietary supplements. Zeolites are believed to have detoxifying properties and are used to support overall health and well-being.

Ingredients: Zeolite supplements contain various forms of zeolites, such as clinoptilolite, which are natural mineral compounds formed from volcanic ash and other geological processes. Zeolites have a honeycomb-like structure with pores that can trap and exchange ions, toxins, heavy metals, and other substances.

How to Prepare: Preparing for zeolite supplement use involves selecting a reputable product from a trusted manufacturer and following the recommended dosage instructions provided on the product packaging or as advised by a healthcare provider. It's essential to choose supplements that are free from contaminants and additives and to drink plenty of water to stay hydrated during supplementation.

Dosage: The recommended dosage of zeolite supplements can vary depending on the specific formulation, concentration of zeolites, and individual health needs. Typical doses range from 500 mg to 5000 mg per day, taken with water or another beverage. It's important to follow the dosage instructions carefully and not exceed the recommended dose without consulting with a healthcare provider.

How to Use: Zeolite supplements are typically taken orally with water or another beverage, preferably with meals to enhance absorption. Some supplements may recommend a specific dosing schedule or additional dietary and lifestyle recommendations to support detoxification and overall health. It's essential to take zeolite supplements consistently as part of a daily routine to maximize their potential health benefits.

Side Effects: Zeolite supplements are generally well-tolerated by most people when used as directed, but some individuals may experience side effects such as gastrointestinal upset, nausea, diarrhea, or allergic reactions. Zeolites may also interact with certain medications or have effects on nutrient absorption, so it's important to consult with a healthcare provider before using zeolite supplements, especially if you have underlying health conditions or are taking medications. Pregnant or breastfeeding women and individuals with kidney issues should avoid zeolite supplements. It's also essential to choose supplements from reputable brands with third-party testing and certifications to ensure product quality and purity.

Zesty Salads (with Detoxifying Ingredients):

Definition: Zesty salads with detoxifying ingredients are nutritious and flavorful salads made with fresh, whole ingredients known for their detoxifying properties. These salads are designed to support the body's natural detoxification processes and promote overall health and well-being.

Ingredients: Zesty salads with detoxifying ingredients may include a variety of fresh vegetables, leafy greens, fruits, herbs, seeds, nuts, and protein sources. Common detoxifying ingredients found in these salads may include dark leafy greens (such as kale, spinach, and arugula), cruciferous vegetables (such as broccoli, cabbage, and Brussels sprouts), citrus fruits (such as lemon, lime, and grapefruit), herbs and spices (such as cilantro, parsley, ginger, and turmeric), seeds (such as chia seeds and flaxseeds), and lean protein sources (such as grilled chicken, tofu, or legumes).

How to Prepare: Preparing zesty salads with detoxifying ingredients involves selecting fresh, organic produce and other whole ingredients and combining them in creative and flavorful ways. It's essential to wash and chop vegetables and fruits thoroughly and to prepare any additional components such as salad dressings or protein sources as needed.

Dosage: There isn't a specific dosage for zesty salads with detoxifying ingredients, as it depends on individual preferences, dietary needs, and health goals. Aim to incorporate a variety of detoxifying ingredients into your salads regularly to maximize nutrient intake and support overall health and well-being.

How to Use: To enjoy zesty salads with detoxifying ingredients, start by assembling a base of fresh leafy greens and vegetables in a large salad bowl. Add additional ingredients such as fruits, herbs, seeds, nuts, and protein sources to enhance flavor and nutrition. Experiment with different combinations of ingredients and dressings to create satisfying and nutritious salads that appeal to your taste preferences.

Side Effects: Zesty salads with detoxifying ingredients are generally safe for most people when made with fresh, whole ingredients and consumed as part of a balanced diet. However, some individuals may experience side effects such as digestive upset, bloating, or food sensitivities if they're sensitive to certain ingredients or combinations of foods. It's essential to listen to your body's cues and make adjustments as needed to accommodate any dietary restrictions or preferences. If you have specific health concerns or medical conditions, consult with a healthcare provider or registered dietitian before making significant changes to your diet to ensure it's safe and appropriate for you.

Zinc Supplements:

Definition: Zinc supplements are dietary supplements containing zinc, an essential mineral that plays a crucial role in various bodily functions, including immune function, wound healing, DNA synthesis, and cell division. Zinc supplements are commonly used to support overall health and well-being, particularly for immune system support and maintaining healthy skin, hair, and nails.

Ingredients: Zinc supplements contain various forms of zinc, such as zinc gluconate, zinc citrate, zinc picolinate, or zinc sulfate, as well as other inactive ingredients used to form capsules, tablets, or liquid formulations. It's essential to choose supplements from reputable brands with third-party testing and certifications to ensure product quality and purity.

How to Prepare: Preparing for zinc supplement use involves selecting a high-quality product from a trusted manufacturer and following the recommended dosage instructions provided on the product packaging or as advised by a healthcare provider. It's essential to choose supplements that provide an adequate dose of zinc without exceeding the recommended daily allowance

(RDA) or tolerable upper intake level (UL) to avoid potential side effects.

Dosage: The recommended dosage of zinc supplements can vary depending on individual needs, age, sex, and health status. The RDA for zinc varies by age and sex, ranging from 2 mg to 11 mg per day for adults. Zinc supplements are typically available in doses ranging from 15 mg to 50 mg per serving, taken once daily with a meal to enhance absorption and minimize gastrointestinal upset.

How to Use: Zinc supplements are typically taken orally with water or another beverage, preferably with meals to enhance absorption. It's essential to follow the dosage instructions carefully and not exceed the recommended dose without consulting with a healthcare provider. Zinc supplements can be used as a daily dietary supplement to support overall health and well-being, particularly during times of increased zinc needs, such as pregnancy, lactation, or periods of illness or stress.

Side Effects: Zinc supplements are generally safe for most people when used as directed, but some individuals may experience side effects such as gastrointestinal upset, nausea, vomiting, diarrhea, or metallic taste in the mouth. Long-term use of high-dose zinc supplements may lead to adverse effects such as copper deficiency, impaired immune function, and interference with other minerals' absorption. It's essential to consult with a healthcare provider before starting zinc supplements, especially if you have underlying health conditions, are pregnant or breastfeeding, or are taking medications, to ensure it's safe and appropriate for you.

Zumba (Exercise):

Definition: Zumba is a popular fitness program that combines dance and aerobic exercise elements with Latin music and international rhythms. Created in the 1990s by Colombian dancer and choreographer Alberto "Beto" Pérez, Zumba classes typically involve high-energy dance routines set to upbeat music, designed to provide a fun and effective full-body workout.

Ingredients: Zumba classes require no special equipment or ingredients but may involve various dance and fitness movements inspired by styles such as salsa, merengue, cumbia, reggaeton, hip-hop, and more. Participants may wear comfortable workout clothing and supportive athletic shoes for ease of movement and injury prevention.

How to Prepare: Preparing for a Zumba class involves selecting a suitable class or instructor based on your fitness level, preferences, and availability. It's essential to arrive early to the class to sign in, familiarize yourself with the instructor and studio layout, and warm up properly before starting the workout.

Dosage: The recommended dosage of Zumba exercise can vary depending on individual fitness goals, preferences, and availability of classes. Most Zumba classes last between 45 minutes to an hour and may be attended several times per week for optimal fitness benefits. It's important to listen to your body's cues and pace yourself during class to avoid overexertion or injury.

How to Use: To participate in a Zumba class, simply show up at the designated time and location, dressed in comfortable workout clothing and athletic shoes. Follow along with the instructor's choreographed dance routines and movements, incorporating elements of cardio, strength training, and flexibility exercises. Focus on enjoying the music, having fun, and moving your body to the rhythm of the music.

Side Effects: Zumba is generally safe for most people when practiced with proper technique and under the guidance of a certified instructor. However, some individuals may experience side effects such as muscle soreness, fatigue, or injury if they push themselves too hard or perform movements incorrectly. It's essential to start slowly, listen to your body's cues, and modify movements as needed to suit your fitness level and abilities. If you have underlying health conditions or concerns, consult with a healthcare provider before starting a Zumba program to ensure it's safe and appropriate for you.

Acupuncture:

Definition: Acupuncture is a traditional Chinese medicine practice that involves inserting thin needles into specific points on the body. It's believed to stimulate energy flow, known as qi (pronounced "chee"), and restore balance to the body's systems. It's used to alleviate pain, treat various health conditions, and promote overall wellness.

Ingredients: The ingredients for acupuncture are minimal and primarily involve thin, sterile needles made of stainless steel or other materials.

How to Prepare: Preparing for acupuncture involves ensuring that the needles and the environment are sterile. Practitioners may also conduct a thorough assessment of the patient's health history and current condition to determine the appropriate acupuncture points to target.

Dosage: There isn't a fixed dosage for acupuncture as it varies depending on the condition being treated, the individual's health status, and the practitioner's assessment. Acupuncture sessions may range from a single treatment to multiple sessions over several weeks or months.

How to Use: During an acupuncture session, the practitioner inserts needles into specific points on the body, typically leaving them in place for around 15 to 30 minutes. The needles may be manipulated manually or stimulated with heat or electricity to enhance the therapeutic effect. Some practitioners may also recommend complementary therapies such as herbal supplements or dietary changes to support the acupuncture treatment.

Side Effects: Common side effects of acupuncture are minimal and may include temporary soreness, bruising, or bleeding at the needle insertion sites. In rare cases, more serious side effects such as infection or organ injury may occur, especially if proper sterile procedures are not followed or if the practitioner lacks adequate training. It's essential to seek acupuncture treatment from a qualified and licensed practitioner to minimize risks. Additionally, acupuncture may not be suitable for everyone, particularly those with certain medical conditions or who are pregnant, so it's important to consult with a healthcare provider before undergoing treatment.

Aloe Vera Juice:

Definition: Aloe vera juice is a liquid extracted from the aloe vera plant, known for its medicinal properties and health benefits. It's commonly consumed for its purported digestive, skin-healing, and immune-boosting properties.

Ingredients: Aloe vera juice is primarily composed of the gel-like substance found in the inner leaf of the aloe vera plant. Some commercial preparations may also contain added ingredients such as preservatives, flavorings, or sweeteners.

How to Prepare: Aloe vera juice is typically extracted from the inner fillet of the aloe vera leaf. The leaf is cut open, and the gel is scooped out and blended into a liquid. Commercially available aloe vera juice undergoes processing and may involve filtration and pasteurization to ensure safety and stability.

Dosage: The recommended dosage of aloe vera juice can vary depending on the individual's health goals and tolerance. It's advisable to start with a small amount, such as 1 to 2 ounces per day, and gradually increase as needed. It's essential to follow the manufacturer's instructions or consult with a healthcare provider for personalized guidance.

How to Use: Aloe vera juice can be consumed on its own or mixed with other beverages such as water or juice. Some people prefer to drink it first thing in the morning or before meals to support digestion. It can also be used topically to soothe skin irritation or sunburn.

Side Effects: While aloe vera juice is generally considered safe for most people when consumed in moderation, excessive intake may cause digestive upset, such as diarrhea or abdominal cramping, due to its laxative properties. Long-term use of high doses of aloe vera juice has been associated with potential adverse effects on the liver and kidneys. Individuals with underlying health conditions, such as diabetes or kidney disease, should use aloe vera juice with caution and consult with a healthcare provider before starting regular consumption. Additionally, some people may experience allergic reactions or skin irritation from topical application of aloe vera juice, so it's advisable to perform a patch test before using it extensively.

Bentonite Clay:

Definition: Bentonite clay is a natural clay formed from volcanic ash deposits and is known for its absorbent properties. It's commonly used in skincare, detoxification, and as a digestive supplement.

Ingredients: Bentonite clay is composed primarily of volcanic ash and minerals such as calcium, magnesium, and silica. It's available in powder form.

How to Prepare: To prepare bentonite clay for topical use, mix it with water or other liquid to form a paste. For internal use, it can be mixed with water or added to food or beverages.

Dosage: The dosage of bentonite clay varies depending on its intended use. For internal use, typical doses range from 1 teaspoon to 1 tablespoon mixed with water once or twice daily. It's essential to drink plenty of water when consuming bentonite clay to prevent dehydration and constipation.

How to Use: For skincare, bentonite clay can be applied as a mask to the face or body to absorb excess oil and impurities. It's left on for a few minutes to dry before rinsing off with warm water. Internally, bentonite clay is used as a dietary supplement to support detoxification and digestive health.

Side Effects: While bentonite clay is generally considered safe for topical and internal use, some people may experience mild side effects such as stomach upset or constipation. It's essential to start with a small dose and monitor for any adverse reactions. Long-term or excessive use of bentonite clay internally may lead to mineral deficiencies or bowel obstruction. Pregnant or breastfeeding women and individuals with certain medical conditions should consult with a healthcare provider before using bentonite clay.

Zucchini Noodles (as Part of a Detox Diet):

Definition: Zucchini noodles, also known as "zoodles," are a popular alternative to traditional wheat-based pasta made from spiralized zucchini. They are commonly used as a low-carb, gluten-free, and vegetable-rich substitute for pasta in various dishes, including salads, stir-fries, and pasta dishes.

Ingredients: Zucchini noodles are made from fresh zucchini squash that has been spiralized into long, thin strands resembling spaghetti noodles. They are rich in water, fiber, vitamins (such as vitamin C and vitamin K), minerals (such as potassium and manganese), and antioxidants (such as lutein and zeaxanthin).

How to Prepare: Preparing zucchini noodles involves spiralizing fresh zucchini using a spiralizer or julienne peeler to create long, thin strands. The noodles can be enjoyed raw or lightly cooked by sautéing, steaming, or blanching them for a few minutes until tender but still crisp. Zucchini noodles can be used as a base for various dishes and paired with sauces, proteins, and other vegetables.

Dosage: There isn't a specific dosage for zucchini noodles, as they can be incorporated into meals according to individual preferences and dietary needs. They can be enjoyed as part of a detox diet or any balanced meal plan, providing a nutritious and low-calorie alternative to traditional pasta.

How to Use: Zucchini noodles can be used in place of traditional pasta in a wide range of recipes, including salads, stir-fries, soups, casseroles, and pasta dishes. They can be enjoyed raw or lightly cooked and paired with a variety of sauces, dressings, proteins (such as grilled chicken, shrimp, or tofu), and vegetables to create delicious and nutritious meals.

Side Effects: Zucchini noodles are generally well-tolerated by most people when consumed as part of a balanced diet, but some individuals may experience digestive upset or bloating if they're sensitive to certain types of fiber or have difficulty digesting raw vegetables. It's essential to listen to your body's cues and make adjustments as needed to accommodate any dietary restrictions or preferences. If you have specific health concerns or medical conditions, consult with a healthcare provider or registered dietitian before making significant changes to your diet to ensure it's safe and appropriate for you.

Zyto Scan (Bioenergetic Assessment for Detoxification):

Definition: A Zyto scan is a type of bioenergetic assessment tool used to evaluate the body's energy patterns and identify potential imbalances or stressors that may be impacting health and well-being. It involves using a specialized device called a Zyto scanner to measure subtle changes in skin conductivity in response to digital signatures representing various health parameters.

Ingredients: A Zyto scan requires a Zyto scanner device, which is typically used by healthcare practitioners or wellness professionals trained in bioenergetic testing and analysis. The scanner sends digital signals representing different health parameters to the body, and the response is measured through changes in skin conductivity.

How to Prepare: Preparing for a Zyto scan involves scheduling an appointment with a qualified practitioner trained in bioenergetic assessment and bringing any relevant health information or concerns to discuss during the session. It's essential to be well-hydrated and relaxed during the scan to ensure accurate results.

Dosage: The duration of a Zyto scan session can vary depending on individual needs and the scope of the assessment. A typical session may last between 30 minutes to an hour and may involve scanning specific areas of the body or focusing on particular health concerns or goals.

How to Use: During a Zyto scan session, the practitioner uses the Zyto scanner device to measure the body's response to digital signatures representing various health parameters, such as vitamins, minerals, toxins, pathogens, and emotional stressors. The results of the scan are interpreted to identify potential imbalances or stressors that may be affecting health and to develop personalized recommendations for optimizing wellness and supporting detoxification.

Side Effects: Zyto scanning is generally considered safe and non-invasive, with minimal risk of side effects when performed by a qualified practitioner. However, some individuals may experience temporary skin irritation or discomfort during the scanning process, particularly if they have sensitive skin or allergies to certain materials used in the scanner device. It's essential to communicate openly with the practitioner about any concerns or reactions you may experience during the session and to follow their guidance for maximizing the benefits of bioenergetic assessment and supporting detoxification and overall well-being.

Wheatgrass Shots:

Definition: Wheatgrass shots are concentrated doses of wheatgrass juice, a nutrient-rich liquid extracted from the young shoots of the wheat plant (Triticum aestivum). Wheatgrass is valued for its high nutritional content and is believed to offer various health benefits when consumed as a dietary supplement.

Ingredients: Wheatgrass shots contain freshly pressed wheatgrass juice, typically extracted from young wheatgrass sprouts using a juicer or specialized wheatgrass juicing equipment. Wheatgrass juice is rich in vitamins, minerals, antioxidants, chlorophyll, enzymes, and amino acids.

How to Prepare: Preparing wheatgrass shots involves harvesting fresh wheatgrass sprouts and juicing them to extract the liquid. Some people may choose to grow their own wheatgrass at home using wheatgrass seeds and trays, while others may purchase pre-grown wheatgrass or ready-to-use wheatgrass juice from health food stores or juice bars.

Dosage: The recommended dosage of wheatgrass shots can vary depending on individual preferences and health goals. Some people may choose to consume one or more shots of wheatgrass juice daily as a dietary supplement, while others may incorporate wheatgrass juice into their diet periodically or as needed.

How to Use: To consume wheatgrass shots, drink the freshly pressed wheatgrass juice directly or dilute it with water or another beverage to taste. Some people may find the taste of wheatgrass juice strong or bitter, so diluting it with other liquids can make it more palatable. Wheatgrass shots can be consumed on an empty stomach or with meals, depending on individual preference.

Side Effects: Wheatgrass shots are generally considered safe for most people when consumed in moderation as part of a balanced diet. However, some individuals may experience side effects such as nausea, stomach upset, diarrhea, or allergic reactions, especially if they have sensitivities to wheat or grasses. It's essential to start with small servings of wheatgrass juice and gradually increase intake to assess tolerance and prevent gastrointestinal discomfort. If you have specific health concerns or medical conditions, consult with a healthcare provider before incorporating wheatgrass shots into your diet to ensure it's safe and appropriate for you.

Whole Body Vibration Therapy:

Definition: Whole body vibration therapy (WBVT) is a form of exercise and therapy that involves standing, sitting, or lying on a vibrating platform or device that generates low-frequency vibrations. These vibrations are believed to stimulate muscles, increase circulation, improve flexibility, and enhance overall physical fitness and well-being.

Ingredients: Whole body vibration therapy requires a vibrating platform or device equipped with a motor that generates vibrations at specific frequencies and amplitudes. Some platforms may also include additional features such as adjustable settings, handles for stability, and various vibration patterns.

How to Prepare: Preparing for whole body vibration therapy involves selecting a suitable vibrating platform or device and familiarizing yourself with its operation and safety features. It's essential to start with low-intensity settings and gradually increase the intensity and duration of vibration sessions as tolerated.

Dosage: The recommended dosage of whole body vibration therapy can vary depending on individual fitness levels, health goals, and tolerance to vibration. A typical session may last 10 to 15 minutes, performed several times per week. It's important to listen to your body's cues and adjust the intensity and duration of vibration sessions accordingly.

How to Use: To use whole body vibration therapy, stand, sit, or lie on the vibrating platform or device and adjust the settings to your preferred intensity and frequency of vibration. You can perform various exercises, stretches, or relaxation techniques while on the vibrating platform to target specific muscle groups or areas of the body. It's essential to maintain proper posture, engage core muscles for stability, and avoid excessive movement or strain during vibration sessions.

Side Effects: Whole body vibration therapy is generally considered safe for most people when used appropriately and under supervision, but some individuals may experience side effects such as muscle soreness, fatigue, dizziness, nausea, or aggravation of pre-existing health conditions. It's essential to start with low-intensity settings and gradually increase the intensity and duration of vibration sessions to minimize the risk of adverse effects. If you have underlying health conditions or concerns, consult with a healthcare provider or fitness professional before starting whole body vibration therapy to ensure it's safe and appropriate for you.

Yoga:

Definition: Yoga is a holistic practice that originated in ancient India and encompasses physical postures, breathing exercises, meditation, and relaxation techniques to promote overall health and well-being. It's often practiced for its physical, mental, and spiritual benefits, including increased flexibility, strength, balance, stress reduction, and inner peace.

Ingredients: Yoga practice requires no special equipment or ingredients but may include various elements such as yoga mats, props (such as blocks, straps, and bolsters), comfortable clothing, and a quiet, peaceful environment conducive to practice.

How to Prepare: Preparing for a yoga practice involves setting aside dedicated time and space for practice and selecting a suitable style or sequence of yoga poses based on individual preferences, goals, and skill level. It's essential to choose appropriate yoga poses and modifications to accommodate any physical limitations or injuries and to listen to your body's cues during practice.

Dosage: The recommended dosage of yoga practice can vary depending on individual preferences, goals, and availability. Some people may choose to practice yoga daily for short periods, while others may opt for longer, more intensive sessions several times per week. It's important to find a balance that works for you and to listen to your body's needs for rest and recovery.

How to Use: To practice yoga, start by selecting a quiet, comfortable space free from distractions and set up your yoga mat and any props you may need. Begin with a gentle warm-up or centering practice, such as deep breathing or meditation, before moving into a series of yoga poses (asanas) that target different areas of the body and promote strength, flexibility, and relaxation. Pay attention to your breath, alignment, and sensations in the body as you move through the poses, and modify as needed to suit your individual needs and abilities.

Side Effects: Yoga practice is generally safe for most people when practiced mindfully and with proper technique, but some individuals may experience side effects such as muscle soreness, fatigue, or aggravation of pre-existing injuries or health conditions. It's essential to practice yoga mindfully, listen to your body's cues, and avoid pushing yourself beyond your limits. If you have underlying health concerns or medical conditions, consult with a healthcare provider or certified yoga instructor before starting a yoga practice to ensure it's safe and appropriate for you.

THE END